I0429861

A Dabbler's Guide to Low Carb Gluttony

by Dr. Bob

This book is an update, abridgment, and re-title to
The Killing of a Nation, a book penned by Dr. Bob in 1995.

<u>From "The Killing of a Nation"</u>

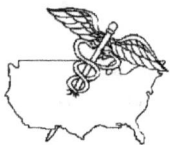

Discover why America's infallible nutritional guidelines
are wrong, and, why America's medical and scientific
communities have a lot to answer for. Discover why
diets are doomed for failure. These disappointments
aside, discover that health and vitality can still be
yours!

Other books by Dr. Bob

I See Bad People: An Introduction to the
Pseudopathic Leader in Corporate America

A Dabbler's Guide to Low Carb Gluttony. Copyright © 2014 by
Robert Allen, Ed.D. All rights reserved.

To my family. You're the best!

Glossary

Preface

The next time you are out in a crowd, make note of the number of overweight men and women around you. You may have to include yourself in the count. The facts are startling. A whopping 69% of American adults are overweight. Their number includes the whopping 35% whom are considered obese. Experts claim that since the 1800s, succeeding generations of Americans have been getting fatter. They don't know why, but they all agree that it is happening. The bottom line is, we have become a fat society.

But, what about our diet craze – this must be having some affect? Not so, say the same experts. The percentage of obese individuals in the overall population has been and continues to be on the rise. Twenty years ago, the prevalence of obesity in America was estimated to be 30%. Ten years before that, it was estimated to be 25%. And so it continues to climb. At any one time, over half of the obese population is dieting. But as more and more Americans fail to lose weight or fail to keep it off, interest in dieting is waning. The bottom line is, diets don't work.

But, what about our nutritional hysteria – surely this must be having some affect? Again, not the case. Even in our most nutritionally-conscious State, California, the percentage of overweight individuals in the overall population continues to grow. Despite eating "healthier", the average American today weighs 20 pounds more than the average American 20 years ago. And the average American 20 years ago weighed 20 pounds more than the average American 20 years before that. The bottom line is, our nutritional guidelines are dead wrong.

Heart disease, cancer, strokes, diabetes, and a host of other obesity-related afflictions have become scourges of modern-day society. Prior to the 1800's, such afflictions were uncommon. Life was shortened by war, famine, disease, and disaster coupled with the unavailability of medical care and the lack of medical know-how ... not by degenerative conditions of dietary origin. Today, heart disease, cancer, strokes, and diabetes remain unyielding contributors to the top seven causes of death in the United States. Much more startling, their incidence is still on the rise. The outlook is not good. And I don't even need to mention health care costs. It is now at a level unbearable to nearly every American. The bottom line is, we are a sickly society.

I'm thinking, *duh*, we must be doing something very wrong. I'm also thinking that America's love of carbohydrates has something to do with it.

<u>DISCLAIMER</u>

I am not a physician, esteemed scientist, registered dietitian, nutritional expert, or legend in my own mind. I am just a simple dude whom for many years battled with weight gain, who eventually recognized the futility of dieting and the gross error of America's nutritional guidelines, and, who could no longer sit back and watch family and friends hurtle down a path of physiological purgatory. I read, listen, observe experience, study, and report. Nothing less. Nothing more.

As with any written material specific to or related to your health, this book is not meant to replace the advice of a medical professional. Don't you dare undertake any weight-loss regimen without first consulting with a physician.

CHAPTER 1

The Shocking Truth About Obesity and Diets

I've made every effort to avoid medical and scientific jargon in my text – which is great for me, since I am but a diet practioner. Where I've found it necessary to include such jargon, I offer simple definitions at the end of the respective chapter.

Three Simple Things

If you've ever read a newspaper or watched TV – which is darn near everybody – you already know what the rules for losing weight are. Eat less, minimize fat intake, and exercise. These three simple things.

Now, it doesn't take a genius to memorize these three simple things. So then why all the diet hoopla?

If it were as easy as it sounds, we would just do it! We wouldn't need more variations of diet books than recipe books, diet empires touting celebrity success stories, supermarkets brimming with every conceivable form of diet food, and exercise fads ranging from the ridiculous to the bizarre. We would just do it! The undeniable truth of it is, these three simple things aren't so simple to more than one out of every three Americans. We know this to be true, because more than one out of three Americans is overweight today. We also know that things aren't getting any better, because twenty years ago this ratio was less than one out of four.

America has been dieting feverishly for over twenty years with no success. It's no wonder our society is flooded with diet books, diet plans, diet foods, and diet gimmicks. There is such a huge market for it, and, demand continues to grow.

Folks, the problem is not you. None of us were meant to be fat. The problem is that we consider these three simple things to be irrefutable fact.

Nothing could be further from the truth.

Fact or Fiction

It's very easy to rationalize the diet mania that surrounds and infiltrates our lives, for after all, America is the land of opportunity (and profiteers). But, not even the experts can explain why America is eating healthier and exercising more – yet growing fatter.

Perhaps we've been asking the wrong people. Let's not ask the fitness guru with the washboard stomach who wouldn't gain a pound if force-fed a thousand Twinkies. Ask an overweight person. I used to be overweight, so I qualify.

Now, I was never gigantic, but I was certainly fat. My weight problems started in my late twenties. To me, it seemed like it just hit. I suppose it actually snuck up on me over a span of a couple years. But even then, I knew what was required to lose weight. Eat less, avoid fat, and exercise. So I did, and I was one of the lucky ones who could actually lose weight. And over the next decade, I lost the same weight over and over and over again. Does this sound familiar to you?

I need to draw your attention to some of the recurring physical symptoms I experienced during my yo-yo dieting years, so permit me to elaborate a bit on how I felt and what I experienced through one of these diet cycles.

While fat, I always felt like a slim person trapped in a pudgy body. I anguished over why I ate less than my thin friends, yet remained fat. I anguished over why I ate sensibly (by published standards), yet remained fat. My bad cholesterol was way high, and my good cholesterol was too low. I lacked energy at times, and I became drowsy after eating. I always seemed to be hungry, even after a meal.

Toward the beginning of my diet, I anguished over why I could eat near to nothing and lose next to nothing. Exercise helped, but it hurt more than I wanted to admit. My bad cholesterol remained high, and my good cholesterol remained low. I still lacked energy, and I still became drowsy after eating. I was always hungry, particularly after a meal.

Well into my diet, I anguished over the amount of time I had to give to exercise and the intensity I had to maintain in order to continue weight loss. At least it didn't hurt that much. But progress seemed agonizingly slow. My bad cholesterol didn't budge, and neither did my good cholesterol. I seemed to have more energy, and I didn't get as drowsy after a meal. I wanted to think that I was finally in control. But the truth was, I continuously thought about food ... what I did eat, what I couldn't eat, what I should eat, and what I would eat.

As I neared my target weight, I felt a great sense of accomplishment, and, felt a great sense of relief knowing that the end was in sight. I almost enjoyed exercise, but I needed to spend more time living. No change to cholesterol. I prayed for the day I could once again start ... well, eating.

With my diet behind me, I wallowed in success and planned for a life ever free of obesity. With great relief, I backed off the exercise. I started to eat a tad bit more, but still much less than my thin friends. I ate wisely, by published standards. And cholesterol – who cared. I had plenty of energy, and I could put up with after-meal drowsiness. I didn't dwell on eating anymore, because now I could deal with it by eating. And soon, I started to feel like a slim person trapped in a pudgy body.

If you were to analyze my personal experiences on the proverbial diet roller-coaster, you would find a pattern of disturbing truths. First, I fought a constant mental and emotional battle – whether fat or thin. Second, effective exercise was punishing and could not realistically be maintained as a lifestyle. Third, I never achieved health and vitality as could be assessed with my cholesterol levels. Last and most profoundly, weight loss was strictly of a temporary nature and could only be achieved in the presence of hunger.

I'll bet that most of you can relate to some of this, and many of you to all of it. The sad part is, there are hundreds of ways to lose weight but none to keep it off. The experts say my story is not unique, because all but an obsessive 3% of those who diet ever really lose weight.

I should consider myself fortunate. With extreme curtailment of nourishment combined with arduous exercise, I could actually achieve significant weight loss (temporary though it may have been). Many of you are not so lucky. Dieting for you means hunger and suffering with little or no weight loss in reward.

Oh, I've heard what the nutritionists and dietitians say about you "tough" cases. You're not trying hard enough or, you're not going about it quite right. So you seek professional guidance to strengthen your resolve and force submission, or, to try a new angle. I venture to say that the lion's share of obese Americans fit this bill, because the diet industry is booming. I'm sorry. America has been there, done that, for the last forty years. We continue to get fatter.

Our society has extensively challenged the three simple rules of dieting with every imaginable tweak and twist. The indicators are clear and undeniable. This is not rocket science. Diets simply don't have any lasting effect.

At risk of offending the throngs of esteemed doctors, scientists, nutritionists, dietitians, and fitness experts who line their pockets with gold on the hysteria and chaos of an overweight and dieting America, I submit to you that only a brainwashed society could embrace today's nutritional guidelines in plain view of our nation's current state of health – particularly when we compare it to that of years past.

The Glucose Factor

It's easy to proclaim that diets don't work, but much harder to explain why. The overweight population knows that those 3-simple-rules of dieting just don't work. The rest and majority of the population insists that they do. The only reasonable explanation, then, must be that some of us were meant to be fat. The fallacy with this is, the fat population is growing faster than the thin population. Soon, the thin population will no longer be a majority.

So why then, don't diets work?

Every one of us knows that we require food as a means to fuel our body. Without food, our body will eventually cease to function. This much is easy to understand. The process of converting food to a substance appropriate to fueling the body, on the other hand, is quite complex. It is unfortunately this conversion process that we must first understand to fully comprehend the ineffectiveness of dieting.

We can group our dietary intake into three basic metabolic categories: fats, proteins, and carbohydrates. As nature has it, the body's selection for energy-use falls in the order of carbohydrates, then fats, then proteins. Most of us know what fat and protein are. Fat is that gelatinous white stuff hanging about a piece of meat, and the rest of it is protein. I am totally surprised, however, at how few can explain what a carbohydrate is. Carbohydrates are a group of organic compounds that include sugars, starches, cellulose (or organic fiber), and gums. Read the nutritional labels on the food products in your cupboard. Most of it consists of carbohydrates. And carbohydrates are wonderful! We can make foodstuffs that don't spoil easily, and, we can produce them in nearly every possible consistency, form, and flavor. And because our medical and scientific communities say so, we know that we must have carbohydrates for energy. Right? Well, I hope to convince you otherwise.

Our body is powered primarily through the use of glucose in the blood. Glucose is often spoken of as "blood sugar". Ingested carbohydrates, fat, and proteins can all become glucose. Carbohydrates most readily, fat less readily, and protein least readily. Now, this doesn't mean that the fuel load is simultaneously shared by all three. With lots of carbohydrates to use, the body basically ignores fats and proteins as a fuel source. We don't want to use protein as a fuel source anyway, because the amino acids derived from protein are the building blocks of muscle tissue. Muscles continuously break down and need to be rebuilt, so thank goodness proteins are last on the fuel preference list. Carbohydrates on the other hand, offer simple sugars which either are themselves glucose or which readily convert to glucose. A quick source of energy indeed! Fat (yuk) breaks down into glycerol and fatty acids. With lots of carbohydrate-derived glucose around, these just become fatty tissue. It's easy to see then why "fat" is such an evil word.

But it is in this very knowledge of our body's metabolic process that a grave misunderstanding lays. The fallacy here is that we consider our body's fuel ranking process to be its most natural and healthful choice as well.

If I introduced a synthetic compound that more easily converted to glucose than even carbohydrates, should this then become our primary source of fuel? Of course not. But, you say, we are not talking about a synthetic compound. We are talking about something that grows from the ground. We are talking about nature's fuel! Okay, so I introduce a supplement in pill-form made from things that grow from the ground that beats the heck out of carbohydrates. You still wouldn't use it, because it would be so "unnatural." What if I told you that carbohydrates, in the massive quantities that we consume them today, are as unnatural to humankind as it gets? Because – nearly all of humankind's existence on mother Earth has been spent with meat, fish, fowl, eggs, berries, and organic roughage as dietary staples. And, I might add, humankind was relatively free of the degenerative diseases that plague modern society.

To believe that humans developed as vegetarians or evolved on a low-fat diet is just silly, ignorant thinking. Only in the last five thousand years did humankind even start to cultivate the land. Only in the last two hundred years did farming take on radically new levels of production as a result of scientific progress, and so, only in the last two hundred years did humankind even start to consume large quantities of refined carbohydrates. Only in the latter half of our century did humankind make refined carbohydrates its primary food source. In the history of humankind, our generation is but a blink of an eye ... not even discernible on the timeline of life. Yet, with all our scientific knowledge and technological genius, our generation has elected to alter humankind's dietary course – making carbohydrates its pill of convenience. The point to be made is that our nutritional needs should not be based on the body's tendency to rank dietary substances as a fuel source. It should be based on the dietary substances that humankind evolved with.

But, enough of history. Whether or not you believe humankind evolved on meat and fish, or pasta and double-layer cake, is not important. What is important is that you understand the metabolic quandary that all dieters face. So let's look a bit closer at our body's mechanisms for fuel consumption.

The Insulin Factor

In order to use glucose to power our body, it must first be processed by a hormone called insulin. Insulin is produced in the pancreas (see the life-like illustration on the next page), which sits in the abdominal cavity below the liver and behind the stomach.

Insulin basically does three things with glucose. First, it stimulates the transfer of glucose to our body's cells for direct energy use. Second, if there is more glucose than necessary to satisfy our cells immediate energy needs, it converts glucose to glycogen which in turn stores in the liver and muscle tissue for future energy needs. Third, if all the stores are filled, it changes excess glucose to triglycerides. It is this last function that is most disturbing. We know triglycerides are "bad" by their common association with high levels of cholesterol. Just like un-used digested fat, triglycerides form fatty tissue.

With this basic understanding of how the food we eat becomes energy for our body, I can begin to explain why so many in our generation are overweight, and, why all the dieting in the world won't help.

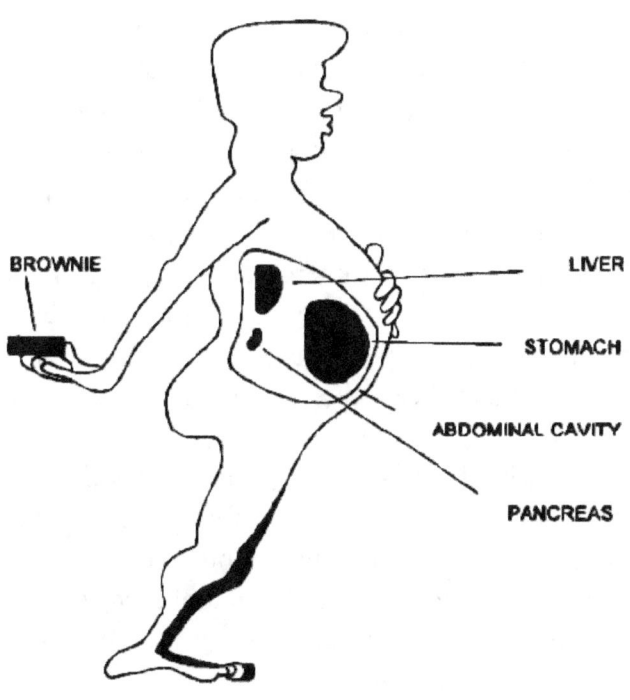

BROWNIE   LIVER

STOMACH

ABDOMINAL CAVITY

PANCREAS

A Formula for Obesity

For the overwhelming majority of overweight Americans, obesity stems from an abnormal metabolic condition fostered by the nutritional guidelines of our nation ... yes, the very same nutritional guidelines meant to assure our health! I must insist that this metabolic condition is not a disorder. Your body is not at fault. You are not to blame.

Our nation's medical and scientific community points us to the inverted pyramid for our nutritional needs. Lots of carbohydrates at the top, much less protein in the middle, and almost no fat at the bottom. We accept this as gospel, because after all, they are the experts. And if absolutely forced to think about it, we could easily assign some sense of logic to it. We need lots of carbohydrates for energy and a bit of protein for muscles – but fat, is simply good for nothing. My friend, from the day you could understand the spoken word, you have been the unwitting victim of poor advice.

For nearly all of humankind, the metabolic traits of our ancestors still dominates. In following our nation's nutritional guidelines, we subject our body to levels of glucose far beyond its natural metabolic capacity. We ask it to use carbohydrates alone for fuel, with a digestive system undeveloped for this task. Unknowingly, we have forced our body into a state completely abnormal to nature.

When you consume a meal or snack of carbohydrates in the massive quantities of today's standards, your blood sugar level jumps. Your pancreas responds, dumping insulin just as fast as it can. The result is, your insulin level escalates rapidly to meet the demand for processing glucose. Here's where that "abnormal metabolic condition" I spoke of comes to bear. The abnormality to our body's metabolic process begins with this tremendous overage of insulin following excessive carbohydrate consumption. This avalanche of insulin in our bloodstream, it turns out, hampers the transfer of glucose to our cells! Truly an ironic situation. The very hormone that was meant to stimulate glucose-use serves instead to overwhelm and block the insulin receptors at the cellular level. The cursed consequence is that more insulin is needed to get the job done. In essence, it becomes a self-defeating operation. As more insulin is secreted, it becomes less and less effective. And if things weren't bad enough, all this insulin begins to process what it recognizes as "excess" glucose into triglycerides. Through no fault of nature, you have become a fat-producing machine!

Nature's Blend

Allow me to digress at this point for the sake of perspective. Remember that incredulous adult overweight-ratio of 69%? Except for the minuscule and negligible few who truly suffer metabolic "disorders" requiring medical treatment, the 69% population of overweight Americans experience this "abnormal metabolic condition" I've just described. And do you know what? The remaining 31% of non-overweight Americans are not free and clear.

Nature provides us with a hardy and efficient metabolic system at birth. "When" it starts to break down – the point where this abnormal metabolic condition sets in – is a function of individual traits of metabolic resilience, and most significantly, the intensity with which we challenge our metabolic capacities.

For those of us already suffering the effects of an exhausted metabolic system, the extent of our obesity is a function of how much efficiency has been lost in our insulin's glucose-processing ability. This varies from individual to individual, which is why we see obesity range from the pleasantly plump to the repulsively rotund.

My generation is lucky, I gather. In my childhood, I don't recall my parents encouraging me to partake of carbohydrates in massive doses and to shun fat. This much came in my young adulthood. My own children's generation is not so lucky. We proudly enforce the advice of society's nutritional scholars – with the best of intentions, of course. The sad result is that one in three children aged 3-17 are overweight, and, this number is on the rise.

The outlook is no better for that 31% of non-overweight Americans. By dictate and choice, this segment continues to overstress nature's metabolic norms with increasing levels of carbohydrates. Slowly and surely, more and more Americans will succumb to pancreatic abuse, and join the ranks of the overweight.

So, is everyone at risk? The answer is, not exactly. For a fortunate few, a gift of heredity or a fluke of nature will provide for a life free of this "abnormal metabolic condition". For them, just a drop of insulin is enough to process any amount of glucose. These metabolic marvels never abuse their pancreas and will never experience elevated levels of insulin in their bloodstream.

Cause or Effect

Up to this point, I have established that many Americans have become fat-producing machines by the very nature of our commitment to society's nutritional guidelines. I have also established that many more can expect to become fat-producing machines at some point in their life if they stay the course of society's nutritional guidelines.

We know now that the root cause is excessive glucose from massive carbohydrate consumption. We know that the effect is gross overproduction of insulin ... a sad consequence of the self-perpetuating loss of insulin efficiency. We know that the eventual result of a stressed metabolic system is obesity. But, my friends, it is not our body's outward physical appearance that should raise concern – because the real crime is being committed inside the body.

I'll bet few of you have ever thought of obesity merely as a symptom. I know I didn't. I always considered obesity to be a cause, a cause for increased risk to heart disease for example. This is simply and sorrowfully a false impression that most Americans hold.

It is true that there is a connection between obesity and many degenerative diseases, including cardiovascular disease, cancer, and diabetes. It is also a matter of fact that a larger percentage of obese individuals suffer degenerative diseases than their slim-and-trim counterparts. But this where the connection ends.

Degenerative diseases are not at all limited to the overweight. Few question why an avid runner or seemingly fit middle-aged individual suffers a heart attack or stroke. A curiosity for sure, but we easily dismiss it as a quirk of fate. The startling truth is that modern-day degenerative diseases – though prevalent in the overweight – afflict all gender, sizes, shapes, ages, and origins of Americans. It is with this fact that we know that obesity is a symptom and not a cause.

The Glucose and Insulin Health Factors

It is important that you understand that glucose and insulin are both natural and necessary components of metabolic vitality. It is even more important that you realize that an excess of glucose and insulin bear much of the blame for the big hitters of today's life-threatening diseases, namely:

Cardiovascular Disease
Cancer
Diabetes
High Blood Pressure

Elevated levels of glucose and insulin also factor heavily into many "lesser" health ills and discomforts of modern-day society, including:

Gall Bladder Disease
Liver Disease
Kidney Disease
Colitis
Ulcers
Chronic Constipation
Chronic Diarrhea
Gas and Bloating
Sleep Disorders
Recurring Headaches
Mood Swings
Depression
Irritability
Anxiety
Loss of Concentration
Loss of Mental Acuity

If you are among the ranks of 225 million overweight adults in America, many of these "lesser" items may already be an accepted fixture of your life. Remember, and be warned, that obesity is a symptom of a metabolic system gone awry. If you are overweight, you indeed possess high levels of glucose and insulin in your bloodstream. Therefore, you also nurture the development of the life-threatening diseases listed.

But, this chapter is meant to offer insight to obesity and diets. So the specific relationships of glucose and insulin to the listed diseases and ailments are further discussed in Chapter 5. What I do need to mention at this point is that, for the 85 million Americans who are not overweight, this is your list too. Only a small fraction of your ranks are the metabolic marvels that I previously spoke of (that is, those individuals who will never in their lifetime experience elevated levels of glucose and insulin). The rest of you, as a result of continuous and excessive carbohydrate consumption, are at some progressive stage of metabolic deterioration. You are at a point where the fat-producing insulin machine (that is, the loss of insulin efficiency) has not yet developed beyond your body's rate of energy use. So, the fat-saving process never really kicks in. But unfortunately, your glucose levels remain higher for longer periods of time than for our metabolic marvels, and, your insulin levels spike where our metabolic marvels' don't. For you, glucose and insulin are hidden evils, stalking you like a killer in the night. We know this to be true, because the diseases and ailments that I list – again, though prevalent in the obese – hardly spare the thin. A profound example of these processes at work in the non-overweight can be found with research in the way of autopsies performed on recently deceased children and young adults of normal weight. Alarmingly, atherosclerosis (or, the buildup of plaque within a blood vessel) was already at play in many of them.

The overweight know beyond a shadow of a doubt they are at extreme risk. The non-overweight of "gifted" metabolic function are at little to no risk. The non-overweight situated at or progressing through some stage of reduced insulin efficiency bear a risk factor somewhere between the overweight and the metabolically gifted. If you are not overweight, the sixty-four thousand dollar question is ... which category of non-overweight are you?

The Glucose and Insulin Diet Factors

Assuming you've not thumbed directly to this page, you should now have some level of understanding about the decisive and devious role both glucose and insulin play with obesity. Yet two questions still remain. Why is it so difficult to lose weight, and, why is it virtually impossible to keep it off?

The pragmatic answer (and my choice of response) is that our society's nutritional guidelines simply won't allow it. The compelling answer, however, requires one last look at the self-incarcerating processes which result from elevated glucose levels, and subsequently, elevated insulin levels.

First and least significant, insulin in excess doesn't do our brain any favors. A spike of insulin, it seems, tends to suppress various neurological functions of the brain. The very noticeable effect is, we get drowsy soon after consuming a meal high in carbohydrates. The immediate countermeasure is to increase motor activity, whether it be shaking the head or getting up and moving about. Based on what most Americans believe to be the perfect source of energy, another countermeasure would be to revive ourselves on yet more carbohydrates. A malicious cycle transpires. But wait, you say. What about all those thin individuals who also do the head bobbing routine after a meal. And again I ask the thin population of America, are you a metabolic marvel, or does your insulin spike?

Second and of substantially greater significance, excess insulin is a breeding ground for fatigue. Tiredness develops simply from the reduced ability of insulin to convert glucose to energy. Fatigue rolls in like an invading army when the astronomically high levels of insulin, through insulin's fat-producing mechanism, eventually drops the body's level of glucose too fast, too much. In medical jargon, this is reactive hypoglycemia. The irony of all of this is that the very glucose that we hope to derive energy from instead serves to inhibit, and then deprive, our body of energy. By today's standards, the nutritionally correct countermeasure would be to search for energy in the way of more carbohydrates. And the malicious cycle strengthens.

Last and most profoundly, excess insulin creates hunger. Research has found that hunger is not a mere factor of how much food we have in our stomach, it is predominantly a factor of how much insulin we have coursing through our body. This much certainly answers one of the many questions I had when I was overweight. Why, it seemed, I could eat to absolute capacity and be hungry five minutes later. If you have any doubts about this stated effect, I would direct your attention to studies aimed at self-imposed starvation. As it is, the sensation of hunger all but disappears following approximately 2 days of starvation. The absence of hunger, in fact, is so prevalent that unless someone interjects, the individual is truly capable of starving to death. The 2-day part is most telling, because this equates to the basic amount of glycogen stored in the liver. Once exhausted, insulin levels drop and stabilize. The significance of this third effect of insulin to diets goes without saying. Diets structured around today's nutritional guidelines never rid you of excess carbohydrates, so the sensation of hunger rarely subsides and strikes hard with the completion of every meal.

Diets Don't Work Because

Many "experts" are finally admitting to the fact that diets fail miserably in the long run. Their explanations for the inevitable return to obesity, however, leaves much to be desired. None ever really set off any logic lights or alarms. And most discouragingly, the blame always seems to land back in the lap of the dieter.

I hope to cast aside any uncertainties you may have about why diets fail. As I ramble through my explanation, I ask you to keep in mind the previously-discussed factors of carbohydrates, glucose, and insulin, and the "abnormal metabolic condition" inherent to obesity.

If I were to identify the components of diet failure by their physiological symptoms and then list them by successive stages of likely occurrence, it would look something like this:

Stage 1.   Diets fail because of the absence or slowness of weight loss.

Stage 2.   Diets fail because of the unbearable physical, emotional, and mental stresses involved.

Stage 3.   Diets fail because lost weight invariably returns.

Let's look at Stage 1. For many of the overweight, employing the three-simple-rules of dieting yields next to nothing in terms of weight loss. In such cases, any diet is bound to be short-lived simply on the perception of futility. For others, employing the three-simple-rules of dieting yields results – but ever so slow. Many diets of this scenario are also short-lived, but for reasons of frustration. The cause for the absence of weight loss and the slowness of weight loss are actually one in the same. Continued carbohydrate consumption keeps your body in an abnormal metabolic state, or better stated, in its fat-producing mode. As a simple matter of fact, the only way weight loss can occur (other than by water loss or muscle-tissue loss) is by forcing the body to burn its existing fat stores for energy. This concept shouldn't be difficult to grasp. In order to get rid of fat, we must use fat. The extent of weight-loss resistance is merely a factor of each individual's acquired level of metabolic dysfunction. Even for the most severe cases, weight loss can be initiated and accelerated by carrying the three-simple-rules of dieting to extremes. This often equates to near-starvation in combination with copious and arduous exercise. So with obsessive resolve, you can indeed overcome Stage 1.

Let's go then to Stage 2. The observation of continued weight loss is the only thing that keeps you going. The price to pay is an unmerciful and unrelenting battle with your physical limitations, emotional capacities, and mental stamina. With your weight dropping, physical strain can actually diminish, though exercise duration and intensity cannot be reduced without compromise to your aspired rate of weight loss. The emotional and mental ride, on the other hand, only seems to get worse with time. The underlying reason is the recurrence of hunger. During periods when you are burning your fat stores, insulin levels are where nature intended them to be. The result is – no hunger. But eat you must. And guess what happens when you eat that banana in corn flakes and milk, when you reward yourself with an extra helping of reduced-fat fettucini, or when you start increasing the size of your regular servings as you climb down the weight-loss ladder? Your insulin spikes, and the gnawing sensation of hunger returns. Each of us bears a different level of tolerance for hunger. For some, it is but one day. For others, it may be one year. To exacerbate problems, we live in a fast-paced society which specifically caters to a carbohydrate-feeding population at every turn at any time. The persistence of hunger coupled with the hysteria of our society's carbohydrate frenzy often becomes an overwhelming force. For so, so many, this becomes the stage for failure. But with the tolerance of Job, a few actually weather Stage 2.

Stage 3 then, marks the beginning of the end. With your target in near sight or, with your weight-loss goal accomplished, common sense suggests that exercise be tapered down and nutritional intake be tapered up. This is the logical purpose of a "maintenance" plan. But unbeknownst to you, any maintenance plan structured around today's nutritional standards is a start-switch for that metabolic fat-producing machine. In the presence of carbohydrates as a staple of consumption, there is no happy medium. You are either in an abnormal metabolic condition, or, free of an abnormal metabolic condition. The switch is either on or off – nature does not provide for a dimmer mechanism. Over the duration of your diet, you were able to keep this switch off more often than not. The extreme reduction in food intake and the extreme levels of physical activity provided for this. The intermittency of this on-again off-again cycle was dictated by a running balance of your glucose-use against your glucose-supply. And all but the most obsessive of dieters make this fateful change from the low-consumption high-activity regimen of a diet to the higher-consumption lower-activity regimen of a maintenance plan. It is after all, an escape from fanaticism and a return to normalcy. Unfortunately, it also re-introduces the hellish return to obesity.

Three axioms for failure and, any one will do. The futility of dieting becomes all too clear.   Diets   fail in the short-term because the abnormal metabolic process of using society's chosen energy source (i.e., carbohydrates) fights you every step of the way. Diets fail short of completion because the abnormal metabolic process of using society's energy source of doctrine (i.e., carbohydrates) overcomes your tolerance for hunger.   Diets fail in the long-run because the abnormal   metabolic   process   of   using   society's nutritional sacrament (i.e., carbohydrates) always leads to the rapid return of lost weight.

Any way you slice it, diets don't work.

Duped But Not Doomed

I admit that I paint a pretty discouraging picture about diets. My experiential evidence demands that I do so. Where our nation's medical and scientific health communities have failed us with erroneous nutritional advice, I have no intention of reserving comment or withholding opinion of blame.

Judgment aside, I am happy to say that nature has not forsaken the likes of you and me. We don't, in fact, writhe in death's grip without hope for escape. There is a solution – so simple, so effective, so natural, so valid – yet so different when measured against our society's twisted perspective of nutritional logic. But real it is, and I and many of my family and friends are a testament to its truth.

If, at this point in your reading, you are convinced enough, confused enough, curious enough, or excited enough, to forego any further discussion of a brainwashed society being led down a path of physiological hardships, disease, and untimely death ... skip to Chapter 3. There you will find what I consider to be our only chance of escape from obesity, and most importantly, from the life-threatening ravages of excessive glucose and excessive insulin. But if you want more mud slinging, Chapter 2 is for you.

Chapter 1 Definitions

1. **glucose**   A form of sugar produced by the body and used as an energy source.

2. **metabolism**   The physical and chemical processes of our body that are necessary for life.

3. **obesity**   By common health standards, an individual is obese when their weight exceeds 20% of the maximum weight considered appropriate for their height.

CHAPTER 2

The Confusion in the Medical and Scientific Health Communities

With every facet of society and its mega-billion$ nutrition, exercise, and diet industries working against me, it goes without saying that I must be as compelling as I possibly can. In this chapter, I offer both simple arguments and unblemished scientific data in support of my "slanderous" dietary convictions. All said, I hope to shed rationale and perspective on the nutritional holocaust I insist exists.

Conditioned for Confusion

I am continuously amazed by the endless procession of ambiguous, contradictory, and conflicting data filing out from the medical and scientific health sectors. For every nutritional study conducted, there always seems to be a second study to refute it.

Case in point. For many years, reports from the medical community stressed the importance of a low-fat diet in improving one's odds in the fight against breast cancer. Then along came a most bewildering announcement in 1992. A huge study conducted by the Harvard School of Public Health found absolutely no relationship between fat intake and the incidence of breast cancer. Scientists since have been scrambling to conduct additional studies to identify the flaws that must exist in the Harvard study.

I'll bet a dollar to a doughnut that most of you can't even recall this study, though you probably heard mention of it when it was first released. This isn't so surprising, because our nation has been bombarded with chaotic nutritional advice so much for so long that we have become apathetic to anything new on the subject. We shrug our shoulders, say "that's interesting", and plod along knowing that yet more findings and rebuttals are just around the corner. Unfortunately, while we wait for the next revelation to hit the street, we play it safe by maintaining a low-fat, high-carbohydrate diet.

New Heights of Confusion

The next time you read or hear a breaking news report or finding about nutrition or dieting, pay particular attention to the exact form of prose. Is it definitive, or is it merely suggestive? Most, I'm afraid, use waffling words like "probably, most likely, seems to, may, should," and "could." Part of the problem is many scientists sell half-baked goods to the media. Even some scientists themselves admit this much. Could it be that some of the evasiveness results from the lack of substantive evidential data? Could it be that some of the evasiveness results from the fact that as a research scientist, where there is confusion there is money to be made? Could it be that, in the desire to keep purse strings open for future funding, sensational or (at the least) supportive findings require the use of twisted reasoning? Bite my tongue, but I say that all of these factor into the current state of nutritional confusion to some extent. Whatever the reason, the confusion is reaching new heights of idiocy.

- First, margarine was good. Then, margarine was bad.

- Vitamin-C supplements were first touted as a way to boost the immune system. Next, it was revealed that Vitamin C was only effective at doing this if you down an entire orange tree. Then the word came out that Vitamin-C supplements don't do squat for the immune system.

- First, fish oil was good medicine for the heart. Then, fish oil went back to being fishy-smelling oil.

- At one time, it was considered life-critical to shed excess weight. Then, the word came out that it is better to stay fat than to repeatedly lose and re-gain weight.

- Initially, we were taught to avoid the consumption of cholesterol. Now, we know that the cholesterol content of foods hardly matters because the body manufactures most of what we have anyway. But still avoid it.

- First, oatmeal was thought to reduce the risk of cardiovascular disease. But then, you had to eat bushels of it before this particular effect would occur. Then, rice took the forefront. I don't know what the current grain of the month is.

- We were warned in no uncertain terms that overeating would send us to an early grave. Then we were told that, if you must overeat, do it with carbohydrates.

- I remember when, without exception, all fat was bad. Then came the olive oil theories. Next it was revealed that saturated fats were badder than unsaturated fats. Then it was determined that monounsaturated fats and polyunsaturated fats were not-so-bad bad fats. And those trans-fatty acid fats, they are so b-b-b-b-b-baaaaad.

Even exercise has not escaped the insanity. Running was touted as the best form of exercise, until middle-aged runners started keeling over with the same degenerative afflictions of the non-running world. Then walking was the best form of exercise, because running could be overly strenuous. Better yet, include aerobic movement when you walk. Then came the stairclimbers, ski machines, rowing machines, and contraptions that look like rocking horses from hell. Then studies revealed that middle-aged men who used these machines for 40 minutes three times a week showed no significant weight loss and absolutely no change to blood pressure. So let's go back to running, because that at least helps us lose weight. Mind you, no less than 40 (gulp) miles per week. Because, according to recent studies, this is the minimum mileage required to see any reduction in our blood cholesterol levels.

Perhaps my silly suggestion of eliminating obesity and its related ills by addressing the root cause comes too late. Because thanks to modern technology, we can now fool mother nature with drugs that reduce the absorption of fat, drugs that increase metabolism, drugs that suppress hunger, drugs that block the brain proteins which trigger cravings, and drugs that stimulate the brain proteins which curb cravings. Even imitation fat that simply passes right through the body is now a reality. I say thanks, but no thanks.

The latest nutritional craze has taken the form of higher math. A maximum of 30% of calories should be from fat, and a maximum of 10% of total calories should be from saturated fats. But because fat-counting alone has been proven to be ineffective in reducing body fat, one must also religiously count total calories. And remember, a gram of fat packs a bigger calorie wallop than a gram of protein or carbohydrate. Not too much protein please. And watch for the changes in calorie-burning efficiency as your weight fluctuates. Ready ... calculate.

Wait one, Einstein. Most experts now feel that a 30% fat limit doesn't offer much protection against cancer or heart disease. So please re-calculate, using a new recommendation of 20% fat.

I recall reading a newspaper article a few years back involving a special report on dieting. In it, registered dietitians had received and answered questions from readers about dieting. One exasperated reader asked why, on 900 to 1000 calories a day and frequent exercise for over two years, he had been unable to lose any weight whatsoever. The response from one of the dietitians was that he was eating too little and that this was putting his body in a starvation mode where calories were conserved instead of burned. I could only suppose then, that the solution would be to eat more?

If none of this is the least bit bewildering to you, I doff my cap and bow in humble recognition. What I see is a panel of experts studying, arguing, postulating, and theorizing -- diligently of course – in the wrong direction. I'm happy to say that at least one-fourth of the world's population will not be so ill-advised. With the rapid westernization of our Chinese brethren over the last twenty or so years came the introduction of packaged foods high in starch and sugar. Chinese experts recently reported that 1.5 million new cases of heart disease are being discovered every year. But unlike their American counterparts, Chinese experts blame this startling trend on the change in their diet. My question for our panel of American experts is, with America eating 10% fewer calories now than the America of 100 years ago, why has the prevalence of obesity nearly tripled since then?

See Spot Waddle

Can you think of any animals other than humankind that suffers from obesity? I can think of two right off the bat. Dogs and cats.

What's curious is that obesity only seems to afflict those raised in domestication. Dogs and cats in the wild don't get fat! And I ask, what nutritional differences might we assign to animals in the wild and animals in our homes? Simple. We select foods for our pets, while animals in the wild select foods for themselves.

Thinking back to Chapter 1, it becomes easy to see how the very same abnormal metabolic process that afflicts humankind would also apply to other animal species of predominant carnivorous development.

Read the ingredients on that bag of dry dog or cat food. It's not unlike reading the nutritional label on a box of snack crackers. A lot of filler, which means, a lot of carbohydrates. And just like their well-intentioned masters, pets suffer gas, a host of digestive ailments, cancer, heart disease, diabetes, and the like. But love them we do ... and the veterinarians love us too.

So blindly do we embrace the nutritional advice of our society's experts that – even in plain sight of incriminating similarities of metabolic abnormality -- we force the same madness on other animal species. This, I say, is the epitome of confusion.

Marketplace Illusions

Take a bewildered society influenced by a befuddled panel of experts, mix them with the world's most creative business minds, and you get a rip-roaring market for health and diet goods and services. And what better way to attract customers than with a visual perception of what we aspire for – the perfect body.

I cast no criticism at such advertisement, for after all, this is just smart business. I only wish to comment on how the illusion of such advertisements feeds the confusion of an overweight society.

I'm sure most of you would kill to have that lithe, supple, sinewy body pictured in that exercise-machine or health-club advertisement. Well, don't kid yourself. These are actors and models with a gift of natural beauty – and they have never had a weight problem in their entire life. Remember, there is a population of 85 million non-overweight Americans to draw chiseled-body actors and models from.

If you've ever frequented a health club, you know that what I say is true. Health clubs aren't "get fit" clubs, they are "for the fit" clubs. Of course the overweight show up, but not for long. It is the hard bodies and hard-body gawkers that keep health club establishments alive. And the truth of it is, such individuals could lose their hard body if they stopped intense workouts, but they may never in their lifetime grow fat.

You may have seen a few diet advertisements that cast normally-fat celebrities professing their successes with this product or that diet plan. Once in a while, a "common-folk" gets in on the act. Just give it some time, and they all disappear from sight. We know from Chapter 1 that diets don't work, and, even celebrities are not immune to this fact. You can easily fool the public with actors and models, but you can't hide an individual who returns to obesity.

And with forces such as these continuously titillating our desire to shed weight, it is easy to see how the inevitable failure to do so fosters a personal agenda for anxiety, depression, frustration, and confusion.

Those Tell-All Statistics

When it comes to statistics, I've always been a skeptic. As Mark Twain attributed to Disraeli, there are three kinds of lies – lies, damned lies, and statistics.

I assure you that with what follows, there is simply no room for deception. There is no ambiguous data to manipulate and there are no unwarranted assumptions to hide. This is uncorrupted, raw data compiled by professional organizations with absolutely no reason to be anything but objective.

As I bore you with facts that evidence a nation falling rapidly from nature's grace, I ask that you remember the metabolic chaos fueled by excess glucose and insulin explained in Chapter 1. Could it be more than a mere coincidence that the rapid development of our nation's health epidemic closely followed society's sudden increase in carbohydrate consumption?

Mortality Facts

As recently reported by the U.S. Department of Health and Human Services' Centers for Disease Control and Prevention:

- Heart disease, cancer, strokes, and diabetes accounts for 55% of all deaths in the United States.

- For ages 45-64, cancer is the leading cause of death.

- For ages 65 and older, heart disease is the leading cause of death.

As I review these mortality facts, one predominant thought comes to mind.

Most Americans die from disease-infested organs!

Cardiovascular Disease Facts

As recently reported by the American Heart Association, American College of Cardiology, and other notable heart-related health organizations:

- Cardiovascular disease remains the number one cause of death in the United States.

- Nearly 1 million Americans will die from cardiovascular disease this year.

- Cardiovascular disease will be the cause of death for more than 1 in 3 Americans.

- Approximately 1 in 4 Americans have some form of cardiovascular disease.

- The economic cost of cardiovascular disease to Americans is currently estimated to be almost $450 billion.

These are startling facts for certain. What is most disturbing is that, with the advancements of medicine and science of America, we should be dying of old age – not from degenerative diseases of the heart and its vessels.

The grim fact is, in the United States, someone dies from cardiovascular disease every 34 seconds.

Cancer Facts

As reported by the American Cancer Society, National Cancer Institute, and other notable cancer-related health organizations:

- There were an estimated 1.6 million new cases of cancer in the United States last year.

- The incidence of cancer in the U.S. since 1950 has increased by 44 percent. And, this increase is not restricted to certain age groups. All ages have experienced increases.

- In 1973, cancer accounted for 17.7% of all deaths in the U.S.. By 1991, it had jumped to 23.7%. The prevalence of cancer continues to rise.

What makes cancer so sinister is that our nation's health experts know less about it than cardiovascular disease, so they can't tell us how to prevent its onset or curb its development with any certainty. It goes without saying that the incidence of cancer is higher now than ever before.

Diabetes Facts

As recently reported by the American Diabetes Association and other diabetes-related health organizations:

- About 26 million Americans (8.4% of the population) currently have diabetes.

- Around 2 million Americans aged 20 years or older are newly diagnosed with diabetes each year. Around 19,000 American youth are newly diagnosed with diabetes each year.

- Over 25% of American seniors have diabetes.

- Cardiovascular disease and strokes are 2-4 times more common in diabetics.

- Cardiovascular disease is present in 68% of diabetes-related deaths.

- Diabetes is the leading cause of blindness in adults over age 20.

- Diabetes is the most common cause of end-stage kidney disease.

- Around 18% of pregnancies are affected by the existence of diabetes during the gestation period.

- The prevalence of diabetes in the United States has increased by some 128% since 1988. If this trend continues, as many as 1 in 3 American adults will have diabetes in the year 2050.

I find these particular statistics difficult to wrap my mind around. The explosion of diabetes over the last 40 years should be reason for as much concern as AIDS and breast cancer. All of these are modern-day health problems. The difference is diabetes kills more Americans every year than AIDS and breast cancer combined. The discouraging part of this comparison is that the long-term treatment of diabetes is so effective that little effort is given in researching its cause and preventing its onset. And I say, the relationship of high-carbohydrate consumption to diabetes is as plain as the nose on America's face. But then, why should we believe the studies which show that tribal and third-world cultures experience an outburst of diabetes within years of introduction to the "civilized" dietary habits of the West?

Health Cost Factors

As recently reported by the U.S. Department of Health and Human Services and other health-cost monitoring organizations:

- America's annual health expenditures are nearing an eye-popping 3 *trillion* dollars. This relates to an astounding average of $8,900 per person.

- America's health expenditures recently reached 17.4% of our Gross National Product (GNP) and evidenced the largest one year rise ever recorded.

- Here's where America's personal health-related dollars are currently going; 32% to hospital care, 20% to physician and clinical services, 13% to home, nursing, and other personal care, and 10% to prescription drugs.

If you think America's health cost woes are a result of physicians charging too much – think again. Indeed physicians these days are wealthier, but only because we must visit them more often, receive more tests and diagnostic exams than ever before, and undergo bank-breaking treatment and corrective surgery just to make it beyond middle age.

Don't Confuse the Truth with Facts

These may very well be attention-getting facts, but (you may ask), what is my proof that the abnormal metabolic condition I attest to plays any part in the existence of the modern-day degenerative diseases addressed? I'm afraid I have no proof. But then, life itself is a kaleidoscope of the unknown and the unproven. All I can do is present what data I have, state my experiences and observations, inject my opinions, and pray that you see the compelling indicators which relate these diseases to the carbohydrate-factor which causes weight gain. And in Chapter 5, you will find the issues which fuel my belief that the same metabolic processes responsible for obesity and diet failure are also to blame for the cataclysm of degenerative diseases plaguing modern-day America. I know of only three absolute certainties in life ... the passage of time, taxes, and death. Beyond this, I can only say that there is a whole lot of evidence which suggests that escaping obesity will distance you from these degenerative diseases.

Chapter 2 Definitions

1. **angioplasty**

A procedure in which a catheter with a balloon is passed into a narrowed segment of artery and inflated with purpose of flattening-out fatty deposits.

2. **catheterization**

A process in which a thin tube is introduced into a vein or artery for purposes of examination.

3. **death (or mortality) rate**

The number of deaths for every 100,000 individuals per year.

4. **endarterectomy**

A procedure in which plaque deposits or blood clots are surgically removed.

5. **incidence**

The number of individuals diagnosed with a disease for the first time (new cases) in a given year. Incidence reflects a society's risk of developing the disease.

6. **prevalence**

The total number of individuals known to have a disease at a particular time. Prevalence reflects the disease's burden on society.

7. **stroke**

Descriptive of brain cell damage caused by an insufficient supply of blood to part of the brain.

CHAPTER 3

Your Average Low-Carb Plan

Strap in and hang on to your gut, because here comes the miracle of low carbohydrate consumption. Call it a plan, a regimen, a culinary convention, a nutritional preference, or a lifestyle ... but don't call it a diet. Diets don't work, and I promise you, this does.

Believe It or Not

You may not yet be convinced that our nutritional guidelines are at fault. And I understand, for so strong are the influences of a lifetime of brainwashing. I hope, at the least, that I've planted some seeds of doubt over the direction that our country's state of health is heading. I also hope that you harbor serious doubt as to the effectiveness of dieting.

I trust, however, that you now possess basic knowledge on the factors involved with our body's metabolic function. Good then! We both have the same level of understanding. I can now begin to describe how lowering your daily intake of carbohydrates can help you lose weight and keep it off for good.

We know that for energy, the body uses carbohydrates first, fats second, and proteins last. But did you ever wonder what would happen if we cut out the carbohydrates altogether? Of course not, because what idiot would cut out life's prime and most plentiful source of energy. But I'll ask anyway. What do you suspect would happen? Would we become weak, then dysfunctional, wither away, and die? You may think so, because you know that this is what happens to people who starve. I retort that I am not talking about starving. I am merely stopping carbohydrate intake. For most Americans, this represents a most perplexing question for sure.

My answer to you is, when we all but eliminate carbohydrates, our body returns to its most correct, most efficient, and most healthful metabolic state – and burns fat for fuel. And indeed, this has been a most natural process for generations upon generations of humankind!

Go ahead and laugh ... but please read on.

With one simple experiment, not even the most narrow-minded, stubborn, and defensive scientist could deny the existence of this fat-burning process. The experiment would be, simply, do it. Cut out all (and I mean all) carbohydrates from one's diet for a week or two – but continue to eat protein and fat – and see what happens. It isn't a fluke, it isn't freakish, and it isn't magic. It is the very same process that sustains animals when they hibernate. It is, in fact, the very same process that permits a reduction in body fat when we diet obsessively.

Nature's Norms

If you recall from Chapter 1, I mentioned that our body is fueled primarily with glucose. There is a bit of a misconception in this statement (which I apologize for), but I had no choice. In terms of a nation intent on consuming massive quantities of carbohydrates, this is emphatically true. The misconception is that glucose should be the predominant and most important source of energy. It is, in fact, a necessary component of life, but it is hardly the body's only source of fuel for its cells.

Make no doubt that glucose is essential. Even in starvation, our body still maintains a fairly constant level of blood sugar. For such a drastic scenario, it uses up glycogen stores quickly, then it draws from fat stores, and to a much lesser (but gradually increasing) extent, from muscle tissue itself. Also make no doubt that for the vast majority of Americans, glucose rarely stays at the level nature intended it to be at.

Enter lipolysis, a word which describes the proven process of our body using fat for energy. Glucose, it seems, was only meant by nature to satisfy the rapid-energy needs of certain cells at the immediacy of demand. Beyond this, the process of lipolysis was meant to supply all the rest of the energy. Many cell groups of the body, including that of the brain and our critical organs, work most efficiently on energy derived through lipolysis. When you were dieting and periodically achieved normalcy of glucose levels (when that fat-producing insulin switch was in the "off" position), you were in fact in lipolysis. It was also such times that you felt most vivacious and most alert.

As a result of our country's long-standing decree to worship carbohydrates, you may never have experienced lipolysis in your entire life. A crying shame, because lipolysis is nature's true formula for health and vitality.

Lipolysis is the process nature intended for transition from a breast-feeding baby to a fully-weaned child. But for so many Americans now and past, the ill-advice of a scholarly nation never allowed for this transition. I would love to convince you that low-carbohydrate intake does.

Low Carb Gluttony

There are quite a few low-carb ideologies currently being espoused and even more low-carb "diets" being marketed. It can be a bit befuddling. The good news is – any one of them that truly restricts carb intake below your particular carb-tolerance threshold (... more on that in a bit) will work wonderfully. But if you should ask me to make a recommendation, I would mention the Atkins Plan – if only because that's what I'm most familiar with. You would be in good hands, because there is no higher authority on the science and magic of low carbohydrate consumption than Dr. Robert Atkins.[1] Whatever low-carb plan happens to spark your curiosity or tickle your fancy, find comfort in the fact that they all employ similar design models for weight reduction. If you were to peel away each plan's medical minutia, scientific complexities, and success stories ... they would all involve curtailment of carbohydrates in one's daily diet. Some have very differing opinions on how much to curtail carb intake, and, how to deal with protein and fat in one's daily diet. Suffice it to say that a plan's carb-restriction design is the only factor that you should concern yourself with.

Does this mean that you can never again eat starches like potatoes and rice or sweeter foods like fruits and chocolate? Not hardly (and in Chapters 7 and 8, you will find out why). In fact, we can't really completely avoid carbs when we eat, because even food forms of "pure" protein and fat have trace amounts of carbs. And what little carbs we do consume in this manner is just fine by nature, because the development of humankind's metabolic processes over millions of years handily accepts some level of carbs intake.

The secret is maintaining our carb intake within nature's range of acceptance. By doing this, we in fact prevent the onset of (or in the case of so many

---

1. Dr. Robert Atkins passed away in 2003 at the age of 73 from an accidental fall that resulted in traumatic (and fatal) brain injury. To this day, rumors persist that he died from his own diet. This is an absolute falsehood that continues to thrive on public ignorance, media sensationalism, and an arrogant medical community.

Americans, stop the continuance of) the abnormal metabolic condition stressed in Chapter 1. By doing this, we keep the fat-producing insulin switch in the "off" position. If you want a glimpse of just how demanding a low carb plan is, or just how difficult life would be without excess carbs, thumb to Chapter 6 and take a quick peek at the most rigid segment (the first 2-4 weeks) of the plan.

For the sake of reference, there is a general consensus in the low-carb community that the on-off point for the fat-producing insulin switch is somewhere near 40 grams per 24-hour period. In Chapter 7 you will learn that this varies slightly from individual to individual, and, can even be altered somewhat with exercise. But suffice it to say that 40 grams is nature's average daily tolerance for carbohydrates.

I know that keeping carbs below 40 grams per day may seem a bit drastic to you. You see this as the complete elimination of many foods that are as normal to your life as walking and talking. I'm afraid this is your ill-advised nutritional conscience speaking to you again. Think back to my discussions on the ills of glucose and insulin, and their corruptive affect to weight loss. The evidence is there, and if you are overweight, the evidence is you.

But to quell any immediate uncertainties you may have about how "easy" low-carb plans really are, allow me to explain why compliance is truly so simple, and so tempting as well.

On a low-carb plan, your daily selection of foods will include T-bone steaks, rib roast, sausage, bacon, eggs, salmon, chicken, gravy, butter, and vegetables in rich dressing ... to name a few. In fact, nature's tolerance for non-carbohydrates is so faultless that you can eat these types of foods without fear of overeating, without calorie counting, and without affect to the natural process of weight-loss and weight-stabilization you've just invoked by turning the fat-producing insulin switch to "off".

The truth is, low-carb plans are anything but diets. On a low-carb plan, you literally eat yourself back to the ranks of the non-overweight. But because obesity is just a symptom, the true benefit of low-carb plans reside with their ability to resurrect health and vitality. So I urge you, overweight or not, to make this change. Turn that switch off, perhaps for the first time in your adult life ... and experience the sanctity of a low-carb plan.

Prove It to Yourself

Okay – so these here "low carb plans" may seem entirely incredulous to you right now, but I suggest that the proof is in the pudding. Try the example "starter" plan offered in Chapter 6 ... and be amazed. What do you have to lose? Absolutely nothing – unless you consider 2-4 weeks of gluttony a "loss."

Chapter 3 Definitions

1. **lipolysis**   The body's metabolic process of breaking fat down and using it for energy.

CHAPTER 4

How and Why Low-Carb Plans Work

Imagine.   Weight loss and lifelong weight-stability without calorie counting, fat-gram counting, specially prepared diet foods, liquid foods, diet medication, magic pills, operations, fanatical exercise, tutored support sessions, hypnosis, medication, or voodoo. Discover how easily a low-carb plan can wrest you from the grips of obesity, and why low-carb plans are nothing short of miraculous.

The Ketone Connection

Lipolysis, you've learned, describes the body's most indefectible metabolic process of breaking fat down and using it for energy.   And you've also learned that lipolysis only occurs when our fat-producing insulin switch is in the "off" position (that is, when we keep our carbohydrate intake below an average of 40 grams per day).

If we search within the lipolysis process for the exact chemical substance that – with the fat-producing insulin switch off – replaces glucose as the primary fuel for cells, we find ketone bodies.   Or simply, ketone. When one is experiencing the natural wonderment of lipolysis, the specific process of using ketone for body energy is referred to as "ketosis."   Thus, when we are experiencing lipolysis, we are in fact "in ketosis."   And to be in ketosis is to be in a most energy-efficient and most natural state of metabolic order.

Ketosis Neurosis

To diabetics and many ill-informed physicians and health-care professionals, the word "ketosis" strikes fear at its very mention. Because coincident with diabetes, ketosis spells ketoacidosis – and ketoacidosis means a life-threatening condition. Should a diabetic's glucose level rise precipitously high, they would indeed enter a state of ketosis. The difference between this diabetic and you is, the diabetic's blood sugar is out of control, while yours is very much in control.

To the non-diabetic, ketosis is anything but life-threatening. It is, in fact, life giving to the highest degree.

The Ketosis Weight-Loss Miracle

If you recall from Chapter 3, an individual consuming carbohydrates by today's standard stores approximately 2 days' worth of glycogen in the liver. These reserves, then, must first be used up before ketosis can receive its call to duty.

As it is, from the point one initiates the reduction of daily carbohydrate intake to less than 40 grams, the fat-producing insulin switch remains "on" and ketosis lays dormant until approximately 48 hours have elapsed. Much like as would be observed on a fasting diet, the gnawing sensation of hunger only disappears with the onset of ketosis. The obvious difference between a low-carb plan and a fasting diet is, one eats like a king on the low-carb plan, while one eats not a thing on a fasting diet. So it is easy to see that eating your way into ketosis offers a more desirable approach than fasting your way into ketosis. And as the initial 48 hours of glycogen use draws to an end, the fat-producing insulin switch clicks off -- and ketosis enters the game. The miracle of a low-carb plan can finally begin.

In ketosis, the body must draw from ingested fats and stored fats for energy. And with the body in perfect metabolic balance, a truly remarkable weight-adjustment and weight-regulation process takes place. The body strives to re-establish and then maintain nature's chosen weight ... or should I say, nature's chosen non-overweight weight. The pounds come off steadily, and because of normalized insulin levels, all in the absence of hunger. The icing on the cake is the way you feel. The combination of controlled levels of glucose and insulin coupled with a most perfect source of fuel (in the way of ketone) rewards you with new-found energy, emotional stability, and alertness.

During the few days following the tremendous drop in insulin levels (at the onset of ketosis), you may experience a sudden and significant reduction in weight. Much of this immediate weight loss is simply water loss – that is, extra water that you have been carrying needlessly for ages. It is no secret that insulin tends to increase both salt and water retention. The sudden drop of insulin to nature's intended level, as such, brings with it a diuretic affect.

It is also worthwhile mentioning that eating your way through weight reduction is so very much healthier than fasting your way through weight reduction. The absence of food intake spells a critical shortage of many essential nutrients and vitamins, and the effects can be undesirable and often dangerous. Fasting also bears the distinction of burning protein as well as fat for energy. And to muscle tissue, this is hardly an ideal situation. A low-carb plan, in fact, is so metabolically flawless that weight loss can actually occur faster than would be observed during a fast.

With ketosis in full swing, obesity flees your body with every bite of mouth-watering steak, and with every gulp of butter-fried egg. And were you still following the erroneous advice of our nation, this same number of calories would be packing the weight on hand over foot. On a low-carb plan, the calorie-to-weight theory taught by nutritional experts and espoused by our society is seen for a sham. The self-regulating mechanism inherent to ketosis leaves no doubt to this. Because regardless of the amount of protein-calories and fat-calories consumed while in ketosis, excess weight continues to disappear. And regardless of the amount of protein-calories and fat-calories consumed after your weight has stabilized at nature's ideal, weight gain does not occur. So perfect is ketosis that unused calories in the form of ketone is simply liberated from the body in the urine, and to a lesser extent, from the tongue. And with this process of ketone liberation comes a most convenient method of monitoring the position of that fat-producing insulin switch.

Because diabetics must concern themselves with the presence of ketone (and ketoacidosis), urinalysis strips

– commonly called ketostix – are readily available on the market which accurately measure ketone production. With these test strips, the issue of approximating your particular carbohydrate threshold goes away. With a simple 15-second ketostix test, we can easily narrow down the individual value of carbohydrate grams we must remain under on a daily basis in order to keep the fat-producing insulin switch in the "off" position.

Obesity Tried, Convicted, and Exiled

When we relate the near-magical effects of ketosis to the three axioms of diet failure discussed in Chapter 1, it becomes all too clear why low-carb plans work so well – and work utterly alone – in reducing weight and keeping it off.

In ketosis, the body's most natural process of burning fat for fuel assures us weight loss. Immediate and constant. No sense of futility. No sense of frustration. And lots and lots of food. Strike Stage 1 as a factor for failure.

In ketosis, the stabilization of insulin equates to the complete absence of hunger. Immediate and constant. No emotional and mental turmoil. And lots and lots of food. Strike Stage 2 as a factor for failure.

In ketosis, no change to physical activity or caloric intake follows the completion of weight loss. The fat-producing insulin switch remains off. And lots and lots of food. Strike Stage 3 as a factor for failure.

With the birth of ketosis comes the everlasting expulsion of obesity from your life. I challenge you to bring obesity to justice with a low-carb plan!

Factors of Reduced Efficiency

For every rule, there is always an exception. And so it goes with the claimed effectiveness of a low-carb plan.

For an extremely small percentage of the overweight, various factors may yield less than gratifying results unless special measures are taken. But don't fret. With the simplest of adjustments, the miracle of low-carb plans are still yours for the taking.

Extreme Metabolic Resistance

Following the first 2 full days on a customary low-carb plan, your body should be in ketosis. The ketostix test will tell. If you find that you are not, continue eating the foods allowed by the 2-4 week menu (see Chapter 6) except reduce the carbohydrate-containing foods to a level well below the 40 gram per day mark. Find out what daily level of carbohydrate intake shuts that fat-producing insulin switch off for you. 20 grams per day may do it. For some, it may require 10 grams or less. For the severely metabolic resistant, ketosis may only come with the near absence of carbohydrates in the diet. But come it will. Even in the most profound of cases, a combination of extreme carbohydrate restriction and exercise (which, you will learn in Chapter 7, serves to nudge the body's carbohydrate tolerance upwards) will bring ketosis about.

Food Intolerances

Should you find yourself well in ketosis but experiencing little weight loss, you may be the victim of a specific intolerance to a food. In general, such intolerances fall into a category of a yeast intolerance or an allergy-based intolerance. Yeast intolerances are often characterized by gas, bloating, sweet cravings, and chronic constipation. Prolonged use of certain medications, and, other subtle influences to a weakened immune system are often to blame for the development of a yeast intolerance. If you suspect that a yeast intolerance is at play, the simple solution is to minimize or eliminate yeasty foods typically allowed on the a low-carb plan – such as cheese, fermented condiments, vinegar, fermented beverages, and yeast-risen breads. Allergy-based intolerances are often characterized by headaches, mental lethargy, and diarrhea. Much like allergies to pollens, dust, or insect stings, allergic reactions to food groups vary from individual to individual. Low carb foods most typical to a digestive allergic response include eggs, cheese, tomatoes, beef, chicken, onions, coffee, and artificial sweeteners. If you suspect that an allergy-based intolerance is at play, elimination may require some personal experimentation. Make note of the foods eaten just prior to the onset of what you consider to be an allergic reaction. Isolate foods of likely cause and cut them from your diet. Reintroduce suspect foods one at a time and observe for allergic response. In time, you will know precisely which foods prompt the allergy.

In both yeast intolerances and allergy-based intolerances, the elimination of "culprit" foods brings quick relief from the annoying discomforts that often accompany the intolerance, and, brings a notable increase in the rate of weight loss.

Again, I mention these factors of reduced weight-loss efficiency simply because they exist. But remember, for the vast majority of overweight individuals who (most wisely) undertake a low-carb plan, no special considerations of food intake are required to experience constant weight loss, and, the normalizing action of ketosis alone is enough to rid you of any intolerance-like discomforts.

Words of Caution for Two

I can think of two cases where a low-carb plan may not be appropriate for you, and could very well be dangerous to you, without close supervision by a physician both knowledgeable in the metabolic processes of the body and familiar with the metabolic changes that a low-carb plan will most certainly effect. These are individuals who suffer from diseases of digestive organs such as the gall-bladder, liver, and kidneys, and, individuals with diabetes (both Type I and Type II). Where irreversible damage to the digestive system has already occurred, nature's components for metabolic normalcy are no longer intact. The sad truth is, a lifetime of excessive carbohydrate intake was most likely a factor in the development of your condition. And now, carbohydrates may present your most compatible choice of foods. Never your healthiest, but perhaps your most compatible.

If you fit one of these categories, take heart. I am not saying that you will never be able to use a low-carb plan and experience its weight-loss effectiveness. I am saying that your condition presents unique risk factors that should only be challenged by a medical professional. Diabetics offer the simplest example of such risks. Because low-carb plans severely restrict carbohydrate intake (duh), failure to adjust insulin intake accordingly could have dire consequences. But because a low-carb plan substantially reduces the body's insulin demand and serves to stabilize glucose levels, diabetics also stand to gain the most from its use.

As a diabetic, your task will be to find a physician willing to undertake a dietary convention entirely opposite to what is taught to be "correct."

Go and Sin No More

It always upsets me to think of the many years I fought vigorously against weight gain – when all along it was but a simple matter of turning the fat-producing insulin switch off. So easy, so painless, so logical, and so well-hidden among the fallacies of modern-day nutritional guidance.

You may be reading this book because you are overweight and frustrated, concerned about your health or someone else's health, simply interested in all things nutrition, or feel obligated to do so after I forced it on you. In any case, you have absolutely nothing to lose and everything to gain by trying it. The nutritional sins of society weigh heavily on your mind, soul, ... and body. Redeem yourself with a low-carb plan.

Look to Chapter 6 for examples on starting a low-carb plan. Once finished (and thoroughly amazed) with the initial 2-4 weeks on any plan, Chapter 7 can guide you through continued weight loss and a life free of obesity.

Chapter 4 Definitions

1. **allergy**   Abnormally high physical sensitivity to certain substances.

2. **calorie**   A unit measure of a food's energy-producing potential roughly equal to the amount of heat required to raise the temperature of 1 kilogram of water by 1°C.

3. **diuretic**   Tending to increase the discharge of urine.

4. **ketoacidosis**   A life-threatening condition unique to diabetics resulting from out-of-control glucose levels.

5. **ketone**   An organic hydrocarbon compound (of the same class as acetone) produced by the body.

6. **ketosis**   A normal metabolic condition involving the body's production of ketone, and its subsequent use as cell energy.

7. **yeast**   An agent capable of fermenting carbohydrates.

CHAPTER 5

Health and Vitality with a Low-Carb Lifestyle

The initial wonderment of a low-carb plan comes with its remarkable effectiveness in reducing weight and keeping it off. Its true wonderment, however, manifests with its natural process of removing the root cause for so many modern-day degenerative diseases and "common" ailments. Follow me to health and vitality.

The Thought of Disease Sickens Me

Though I can assure you that any low-carb plan is dieter's heaven, I cannot tell you that they represent a panacea for society's every health ill. I am convinced, however, that many of the health ills of dietary origin common to modern-day America can be prevented with a low-carb plan.

Toward the end of Chapter 1, I touched on both life-threatening degenerative diseases and "lesser" ailments that I say bear strong relation to an excess of glucose and insulin in the body. I offer further explanation to this charge in sections to follow, and hope to bring to view the logic of a low-carb plan in disease prevention and reversal.

Cardiovascular Disease

"Cardiovascular disease" groups an array of functional disorders involving the heart and the many pathways of blood flow. Heart disease alone accounted for one-third of all deaths in our country last year. Now, I'm not talking about an individual dying in old age as a result of an old heart. I am talking about a heart that malfunctions or stops because it is affected by disease. When we add strokes, other forms of blockage, hardening of blood vessels, weakening of blood vessels, and a host of other abnormalities along with heart disease, we have one massive problem on our hands.

Many studies have drawn a clear connection between cardiovascular disease and high LDL cholesterol, high triglycerides, and low HDL cholesterol. Other studies have also associated cardiovascular disease specifically with high levels of insulin (and thus, high levels of glucose). But too few of these researchers have put their notes and findings together, for had they, an undeniable relationship between a high-carbohydrate diet and cardiovascular disease would have surfaced. But then, no researcher in their right mind would dare challenge the veracity of nutritional tenets exhorted by the infallible demigods of medicine and science. It would be the death of their research career, at the least.

As many studies have it, an excess of insulin serves to increase the body's production of LDL cholesterol and to suppress levels of HDL cholesterol. And, as you know, high insulin means high triglycerides. What we have is a sure formula for cardiovascular disease.

On a low-carb plan, your insulin production will drop to nature's intended level – perhaps for the first time in 10, 20, or even 50 years. The result will be a significant increase in HDL cholesterol, a significant decrease in LDL cholesterol, and an enormous decrease in triglycerides. The reward will be protection from the ravages of our nation's No. 1 killer.

It should be apparent to you that I would be a fool to suggest such immense benefit if it weren't true. Because proof is but one simple blood test away. At the onset of any low-carb plan when fat stores are rapidly being used up, total cholesterol may actually increase somewhat. The fact that the drop in LDL cholesterol seems to come slower than the increase in HDL cholesterol doesn't help this initial, but temporary, condition. As a general rule, a cholesterol/triglyceride check somewhere in the vicinity of 2-3 months after starting a low-carb plan should offer a good indicator of the beneficial changes occurring in your body.

Do I believe that a low-carb plan can actually undo an existing condition or level of cardiovascular disease? Yes I do, though I admit that this belief is but blind faith on my part. If what cardiologists say about HDL cholesterol's ability to strip deposits is true, then the significant increase in HDL cholesterol realized through a low-carb plan can only serve as a catalyst for reversal. And twisted though it may sound, I also say that I have a natural solvent coursing through my vascular network. Because ketone is the body's form of acetone. And any mechanic knows that acetone is a most wonderful cleaning solvent. What do you have cleaning your vascular network?

Cancer

Second only to heart disease on the annual death list, cancer represents another scourge of modern society. Let's isolate breast cancer for the sake of example. Women are turning up with breast cancer at a shocking rate of 1 in 8. All told, 3.1 million Americans have breast cancer today. And, this is only breast cancer. Looking at all types of cancers, breast cancer only accounts for 21% of the grand total. These figures are simply astounding. Now, one would think that society's space-age technology would have provided some inkling as to the cause of cancer by now. This unfortunately is not the case. We understand better the mechanisms of cancer once it has set in, and we treat it with greater success, but America is losing the battle to identify its cause.

Perhaps our experts should turn their attention to the findings of a middle century Nobel-prize winning scientist who discovered that, unlike normal cells which feed on oxygen, cancer cells feed on glucose. Let's reflect here ... high carbohydrate intake means high glucose levels means a breeding ground for cancer cells. Straightforward enough for my simple mind.

On a low-carb plan, your glucose levels will always remain within nature's intended range for your cell's immediate energy needs. With the high-carbohydrate demands of today's nutritional guidelines, your glucose levels only intermittently achieved such reductions and stability. And in the absence of excess glucose to cultivate whatever mechanism triggers cancerous growth, protection from our nation's No. 2 killer seems logical enough.

My belief of such protection, much like my belief to the reversal effect of any low-carb plan to cardiovascular disease, requires but another leap of faith. All I can reflect on are those tribal cultures still found today that subsist – as they have for untold centuries – on a staple of meat. For such tribal cultures, cancer is a virtual stranger.

Diabetes

To those of us in America outside the medical profession, diabetes is perhaps the least understood modern-day disease, yet in my opinion, one of our society's most horrific.

Remember the pancreas and how important it is in maintaining metabolic stability in our body? In diabetes, the pancreas exhausts to a significant point of insulin-production ineffectiveness (Type II diabetes) or stops producing insulin altogether (Type I diabetes). This shouldn't be a surprise to anyone, because America's nutritional guidelines precisely encourage the development of diabetes. The sad truth is, 1 in 10 Americans have some form of diabetes. And, the rate of new cases per year keeps on rising. The tragic part involves our children, where the risk of developing diabetes is higher than any other severe chronic disease of childhood.

Perhaps diabetes escapes an ominous tone because it is easily treated and no longer poses an immediate threat to life. The other side of that coin is that the diabetic is faced with a life of medication or daily needles. This other side also shows that diabetics face a shortened life span as a result of significantly increased risks of cardiovascular disease. The tragedy doesn't end there, because diabetics live with the fear of suffering one or more of a host of ailments which substantially affect the quality of life, such as blindness and neuropathy (the latter of which often requires lower-extremity amputations).

It angers me to think that the medical and scientific community fails to see or chooses to ignore the relationship between diabetes and the high-carbohydrate hysteria that grips our society. They can call me a charlatan if they wish (and I'm sure they will), but I maintain that even the feeblest of minds could not deny this relationship with the facts of diabetic incidence and prevalence standing before them.

On a low-carb plan, protection from the onset of diabetes is all but assured. With the extreme reduction of carbohydrates in our diet, the insulin demand placed on the pancreas goes to near-zilch. A level, in fact, intended by nature. It goes without saying that in the absence of continuous and exhausting abuse, the pancreas will thrive. Just ask our tribal neighbors.

High Blood Pressure

High blood pressure (or hypertension) seems innocent enough, because though 67 million American adults experience it (gulp, that's 1 in 3 adults), they're all healthy ... aren't they? High blood pressure is known in medical circles to be a "silent killer" because it is possible to have high blood pressure for many years without knowing it and, because few realize that high blood pressure is a high-risk precursor to heart disease and strokes. We know that heart disease and strokes kill us, but we forget that high blood pressure plays a pivotal role in their development.

It should be simple enough for us to understand the fundamental ills of high blood pressure. The heart has to work harder than normal, and this puts a strain on both the heart and the arteries. What seems to befuddle scientists is exactly why we experience it. The fact is, in 90 to 95% of high blood pressure cases, the cause is unknown. But, not to worry. There are a host of both non-drug and drug treatments that are effective in treating this disease. They include diuretics, beta blockers, sympathetic nerve inhibitors, vasodilators, angiotensin converting enzyme inhibitors, calcium antagonists, and many others I can't spell or pronounce. But they all seem to work and they make us feel pretty secure. High blood pressure, I'm afraid, is another prime example where we treat the symptoms so well that it suppresses the need to find and eliminate the cause.

More than a few scientists have linked high blood pressure with high insulin levels. And, this makes sense. We know that in the metabolically intolerant, excessive glucose spawns high levels of insulin. We understand why high insulin levels are a recipe for fat production and obesity. Researchers tell us that high blood pressure is overwhelmingly predominant in the obese. It all adds up.

On a low-carb plan, an individual without high blood pressure is unlikely to ever develop it. And for the individual already afflicted with high blood pressure of unknown origin (i.e., other than for a known physical abnormality such as a kidney or adrenal gland problem), a low-carb plan is a sure-fire way to treat it for life.

Much like my claim to any low-carb plan's effectiveness in lowering LDL cholesterol and triglycerides, and increasing HDL cholesterol, I have no obscurities to hide behind with my stated effect to high blood pressure. You will eventually find this to be true, because you will see it happen.

Ailments of the Digestive Organs and Tract

As explained in Chapter 1, a diet rich in carbohydrates results in a metabolic system gone mad. Unfortunately, no part of the digestive system escapes this madness. Because cardiovascular disease and cancer pose an immediate threat to life, they are attention-getting and are well suited for statistical comparisons. Less apparent are the ailments which may take a lifetime to kill you, or which are merely cause for discomfort.

At the critical end of such afflictions are gall bladder disease, liver disease, and kidney disease. At the lesser end are colitis, urinary tract disorders, ulcers, diarrhea, constipation, gas, bloating, and sweet cravings. The process of development for ailments of the digestive organs and tract include the repeated or continuous imbalance of organ function, specific food-group intolerances, and the loss of bacterial equilibrium in the intestines – all of which are readily traceable to the metabolic upheavals of carbohydrate digestion. Could carbohydrates be the reason dogs and cats suffer these very same ailments in domestication, but not in the wild?

On a low-carb plan, a cured and calm metabolic system serves to prevent the progressive development of such critical ailments, and, to rid you of the digestive discomforts that you may have already accepted as a fixture in your life. For the ailments of disease, I cannot offer any proof to this conviction. For the ailments of discomfort, my personal experiences are the basis for my conviction. I say, let the elimination of these discomforts from your life form the basis of truth for you.

Ailments of Mental Function

Can you believe that a metabolic system gone mad can actually make you mad? Well I can, because my own experiences say so.

From Chapter 1, we know that glucose is one form of cell fuel. From Chapters 3 and 4, we know that ketone is another (and better) form of cell fuel. Studies have shown that between the two, ketone is by far the best choice for brain function.

Within the metabolic chaos of today's nutritional guidelines, one only fuels the brain on glucose. And if this weren't bad enough, the inevitable swing of glucose levels to extreme lows (subsequent to the massive outpouring of insulin) prompts the body to invoke countermeasures involving adrenalin-like hormone production. The often drastic result of brain cells forced to use glucose for fuel, and subjected to energy-spiking hormones, can be sleep disorders (e.g., light sleep, death sleep, excessive sleep, etc.), headaches, mood swings, depression, irritability, anxiety, loss of concentration, and loss of mental acuity. These ailments sound like a psychiatrist's checklist for admission. And indeed, anyone suffering repeatedly from one or a combination of these ailments may begin to wonder if something more than daily stress or similar influences were at play.

By returning to nature's metabolic norm on a low-carb plan, you can rid yourself of these all-too-common evils that serve to diminish the quality of your life. Immediate proof, simply put, is in its use.

No Room for Doubt

The magical efficiency with which a low-carb plan treats that most telling symptom of abnormal metabolic function – namely, obesity – is enough for me to realize that it truly embodies nature's choice for nutrition. But, for my beliefs that low-carb plans also shield us from society's many degenerative diseases, do I ever experience inklings of incertitude? It would be untruthful of me to say that I never have ... and never will.

Under constant bombardment of health information (affirmed by society's most revered experts) which refutes the sagacity of a low-carb plan at every turn, one can only expect moments of self-questioning. And in such times, I rapidly dispel any seeds of doubt by re-visiting the clear and undeniable facts of Chapter 2.

If I die today of a massive heart attack, is it because of my low-carb ways, or, is it because I failed to use a low-carb plan for the first 30 years of my life? A wise man once told me to temper the advice of physicians with the wisdom of my body. Listen to the way it responds, listen to the way I look, and listen to the way I feel. You would be as wise to question the experts, to listen to your body, and to make your one decisions.

I passionately believe that a low-carb plan is a most powerful chalice of health and vitality. And indeed, I "steak" my life on it.

Chapter 5 Definitions

1. **LDL cholesterol**   Low density lipoprotein cholesterol. Often called "bad" cholesterol, because high levels are associated with an increased risk of cardiovascular disease.

2. **HDL cholesterol**   High density lipoprotein cholesterol. Often called "good" cholesterol, because high levels are associated with a decreased risk of cardiovascular disease.

3. **triglycerides**   A fat found in food or made in the body from carbohydrates.

CHAPTER 6

The First 2-4 Weeks on a Low-Carb Plan

I know where you've been, and I know where you're at. I've experienced the overwhelming feelings of frustration and hopelessness in a seemingly endless fight to lose weight. My war is over, and I am the victor. And in less than a week on a low-carb plan, your body, mind, and spirit too could resound with clear evidence of its truth. Join me in triumph!

Prepare for Success

Low-carb plans are so utterly simple and effective that there are truly no prerequisites to their success. You needn't throw out all the food in your cupboards, sign a contract of resolution in blood, or meditate all night for spiritual strength. Just get started by preparing yourself a feast fit for a king.

Nonetheless, I do suggest that you consider three simple steps of preparation. First, have your blood chemistry checked before you start. This will establish a point of comparison down the line for LDL cholesterol, HDL cholesterol, and triglycerides. Even in the presence of significant weight loss and other clear physical indications of vitality, the cholesterolaphobic fears bred by society may still lurk in the shadows of your mind. A follow-up check for blood lipids can only serve to dispel ingrained misconceptions of fat and its influence to cholesterol-related disease. If you've had such a check done in the last year or so, you are all set.

Second, if you are on medication that could be stopped or reduced for 2-4 weeks without presenting an immediate threat to your life – do so. Many common medications of long-term use significantly inhibit weight loss, even on a low-carb plan. Such medications force you into the condition of "extreme metabolic resistance" discussed in Chapter 4. And as logic would suggest, do not alter your intake of such medication without first conferring with the prescribing physician. It would not be unrealistic of you to suggest to your physician that, with a low-carb plan, you hope to alleviate or lessen the need for long-term medication. Because low-carb plans are so profound in their affect to so many modern-day ailments and discomforts, your condition of life-long treatment may disappear altogether. The lowering of blood pressure, as an example, is one of the more predictable affects of a low-carb plan. While on the subject of high blood pressure medication, if you happen to be one of millions who take diuretics, stop these before starting a low-carb plan – whether or not you confer with a physician. Because low-carb plans significantly reduce insulin levels in the body, and because insulin factors heavily into salt and water retention, a low-carb plan is, in of itself, a most natural diuretic. So in the case of diuretic medication, its relation to inhibiting weight loss is actually of secondary importance to its possible influence to complications of hydration.

Third and last, purchase a supply of ketostix. Because each of us has a different setpoint for that fat-producing insulin switch, use of ketostix during the first

2-4 weeks on any low-carb plan can be most beneficial. At the least, the daily indication of positive ketone brings with it a satisfying and comforting knowledge that lipolysis is in action. And as you progress beyond the initial 2-4 week menu and introduce foods from the long-term menu of Chapter 8, the use of ketostix can help you define a carbohydrate safe-zone for continued weight loss and eventual weight stability. On the subject of ketostix, I have found no "best" time for administering the test. Though ketone production is most prevalent at night as we sleep, a test at any time of the day should indicate the presence of ketone. Don't concern yourself with the exact color gradient on the test strip. As long as it doesn't read zero ketone, your fat-producing insulin switch is off.

Your 2-4 Week Menu

From Chapter 4, we know that placing the body in ketosis is just a simple matter of restricting carbohydrate intake below an average of 40 grams per day. But because we all bear slightly different thresholds of carbohydrate tolerance (and, because you want to see quick results), the foods listed on the 2-4 week menu are those that can be consumed with little restriction to quantity – and still maintain ketosis.

For the first 2-4 weeks on a low-carb plan, you will likely be challenged with sticking to the foods on this menu religiously, be obsessive in reading labels and counting carbohydrates, and use those ketostix on a daily basis. Why 2-4 weeks? Because it offers a reasonable period for feeling-out the nuances of your body's metabolic function and developing a level of carbohydrate awareness that will allow for the introduction of new foods from the long-term menu. There is truly no law to the 2-4 week time-frame. There are no secrets to weight loss on a low-carb plan. Stay in ketosis, and wonderful things will happen.

Here is your 2-4 week menu. You will find important details on these foods in Chapter 8 under "Foods of Unlimited Quantity" and "Foods of Moderation." Please familiarize yourself with these sections before you begin any low-carb plan.

Meats
Any beef, pork, lamb, fish, seafood (except clams, oysters, scallops, and the like), poultry, fowl, and pressed meats.

Eggs
Any

Cheese
Any

Vegetables
Lettuce, cabbage, carrots, radishes. tomatoes, mushrooms, string beans, celery, watercress, cucumbers, olives, onions, garlic, green peppers, and dill pickles.

Oil
Any

Garnishes, Condiments, and Spreads
Butter, mayonnaise, cream cheese, sour cream, salad dressing, mustard, vinegar, hot sauce, oily gravy, cocktail sauce, soy sauce, tartar sauce, cheese spreads, herbs, and seasoning.

Soups
Bouillon or broth only (no thick soups or noodle soups).

Snacks and Deserts
Pork rinds, sugar-free gelatin, sugar-free chewing gum, and real whipped cream.

Beverages and Beverage Additives:
Water (of course), tea, coffee, diet soda, sugar-free drinks and punch, artificial sweeteners, and heavy or double cream.

Wonderful Expectations

Weigh yourself and get going! In two days time, any inklings of hunger will have passed and the miracle of a low-carb plan will begin to unfold. By day 3, you should be getting positive indication of ketone production on your ketostix test strip.

Eat heartily, drink plenty of fluids, and never look back. Be a slave to the bathroom scale if it pleases you.

Watch both weight and inches disappear effortlessly. Experience new levels of energy and acuity. In 2-3 months, marvel at the cardiovascular fitness your blood chemistry check will reveal. Welcome to a new world of health and vitality!

CHAPTER 7

Continued Weight Loss and Maintenance on a Low-Carb Plan

If you stick to the menu laid out in Chapter 6, you can't help but learn of a low-carb plan's absolute truth, and, of the fallacy in America's nutritional guidelines. Though you can remove the factors which for years have kept your body in an abnormal metabolic state, be advised that you will forever bear the potential for this condition. Just as easily as a low-carb plan rids you of excess weight, any return to the errors of past dietary practices will pack it back on. All it takes is a simple flick of that fat-producing insulin switch. This is why any low-carb plan must not be looked at as a diet. It must be a new way of life ... that is, nature's way of life. So shed any remaining notions that fat is bad and carbohydrates are good. And with this chapter, chart a course for life-long success on a low-carb plan.

A New Life Awaits You

Make the transition from the horribly restrictive (jk) menu of your low-carb plan's first 2-4 weeks to the long-term menu of Chapter 8 when you feel entirely comfortable in doing so. Do it now, do it later, do it never. Remember that there is no law to the 2-4 week time-frame. Don't worry about the food police, they are all at your local doughnut shop savoring scrambled eggs and bacon.

Metabolically, there is no difference between the 2-4 week menu and the long-term menu. Both provide for continued weight loss, both assure you of weight stability for life, and both bear the gifts of health and vitality – because both keep you in ketosis. Continuing your low-carb regimen, then, is as simple as eating, eating more, and eating without guilt.

Where metabolic confusion once ruled, you are now in total command. Where you once accepted obesity as a life-long tenant, you have now locked it out and thrown away the key. Where you once lived to eat, you now eat to live.

Welcome to a whole new and wonderful world!

Staying the Course

As you continue with weight loss on your low-carb lifestyle, you will collect insight on the metabolic nuances of your own body, and gather knowledge of foods and quantities requisite to ketone production. And along the way should you unexpectedly find the fat-producing insulin switch back on (as would be indicated by a negative reading of ketone on a test strip), think about what and how much had been eaten in the previous 24 hours and make the necessary adjustments. Because the long-term menu includes many foods of moderate carbohydrate content, one can easily push the envelope for ketone cessation if such foods are not watched closely. In time, you will get a good feel on where your daily carbohydrate threshold is. And feel free to experiment. Though 40 grams per day is a pretty good average, some of you may find a threshold much higher than this – perhaps upwards of 60 to 70 grams per day. Whatever your threshold, remember that ketosis is the key. Without it, weight loss and weight stability stops, and obesity returns.

Even in the unblemished face of weight loss and, in the elimination of many common disorders and discomforts, shades of doubt may surface now and then to challenge your persuasions. So intense is the daily traffic of nutritional garbage on the information highways, one can only expect as much. If you listen to your body, you will know which road is paved with fiction and which road is paved with fact.

I've found that the indomitable stigma of fat represents a most formidable opponent of this sort. If the fat-consumption issue continues to bother you, take solace in the fact that a low-carb plan is generally on the par with, and can easily be much lower in fat consumption than, standard conventions of diet. Because many carbohydrate-laden staples of society are not themselves free of fat, a dietary routine of their consumption can easily bring in more fat than most would like to admit. On a low-carb plan, there is no hidden fat to deal with. Love it or lump it, the choice is yours. There is such a large selection of delicious foods to choose from that the fat issue is truly not an issue at all.

But then some of you may just not be too keen on fat simply from a standpoint of taste. I would strongly suggest that this is more psychological than anything else, but I will assume for the moment that fat just doesn't tickle your culinary fancy. All I can say (amidst violin music) is, bear with it. You will develop new tastes and forget old ones. Just as certain as your body will experience physical changes, you will also adapt psychologically.

If you are an experienced diet yo-yo'er like me, you are all too familiar with weight-loss plateaus. Even on a low-carb plan, you may again experience this offensive phenomenon. Plateaus, unfortunately, are an inalienable quirk to the process of weight reduction. The difference in approach between conventional diets and the Atkins plan is – on a conventional diet one struggles through the plateau with starvation and extreme exercise, while on a low-carb plan, one sashays through the plateau with plate in hand.

From previous chapters, you may recall the weight-loss anomalies of yeast intolerances, allergy-based intolerances, and certain medications. Should you find yourself merrily in ketosis but seemingly unable to clear what you think is a plateau, give consideration to these classic influences of acute metabolic resistance. Did you recently add a new food to your menu, or, did you recently start a medication? If you think the source of your quagmire is a food, moving beyond the perceived plateau may be a simple matter of avoidance. If you did indeed recently start medication, this is most probably the cause. Finish the term of your medication and move on.

Last and not least, I must remind you to have those blood lipids checked somewhere in the period of 2-3 months after you start a low-carb plan. Even though you know your low-carb plan is for real by the way you look and feel, comparison of test results with those compiled before you started a low-carb plan can only foster additional peace of mind. Let this speak the final truth of a low-carb lifestyle.

Exercise and Vitamins

Unlike conventional diet books, you may have noticed that not once in my previous text have I demanded the use of exercise or spoke of it as a prerequisite to weight loss. Nor will I in text to follow. Simply put, low-carb plans are so effective at weight loss and weight stability that exercise needn't be a factor for success. While still undergoing weight loss on a low-carb plan, it is true that the pace of such loss can be increased with routine exercise. But again, you can do it or leave it. I do it and I encourage it, but only because I enjoy it. If only for its proven aerobic and cardiovascular benefits, exercise just makes good sense.

Exercise also brings with it a most pleasant side effect to your body's carbohydrate threshold. Because glucose is still used by many cells for immediate energy needs, exercise serves to increase the usage-rate of glucose and in turn, allows for a most natural metabolic shift of glucose tolerance. The result is, where 40 grams of carbohydrates in a single day may have turned that fat-producing insulin switch back on, a new threshold of 50 grams per day may be realized with the introduction of routine exercise. These values of course are just examples. The extent of this shift will vary from individual to individual and, will vary by the intensity and duration of exercise. And I advise you, exercise will not cure you of the abnormal metabolic condition inherent to your body. Exercise or not, weight loss and weight stability for you cannot occur without ketosis.

Vitamins are another issue worth mentioning. I take them because I want to, not because I have to. The full spectrum of vitamins and minerals necessary for proper biological function are already seen to by the foods consumed on a low-carb plan. But, I figure that a smidgen more of vitamins and minerals in the way of a supplement can't do me any harm. So if only for this reason, I also recommend moderate consumption of multi-purpose vitamins. And food planner's beware, many contain sugar.

Vacation Time

You will be most pleased to know that once you have completed weight loss and achieved weight stability, your favorite chocolate cream pie is both permitted and encouraged under any low-carb plan – within specific boundaries and with strict limitations. So effective is a low-carb plan that the occasional and finite return to the evils of excessive carbohydrate consumption bear little concern.

"Vacation" from your low-carb plan when you feel excess carbohydrate consumption is socially unavoidable, emotionally or spiritually relevant to a festivity or holiday, or instrumental in avoiding a night in the doghouse. I vacation from my low-carb plan on certain holidays, family birthdays, some dinner invitations, and Super Bowl Sunday.

Now, the absolute and unbendable rule: Vacation for no more than 15 times per year, and, never for more than 48 hours per vacation period.

This rule was not handed to me in the form of a stone tablet from atop a mountain. It just uses good round numbers that allow for most occasions demanding or warranting a return to metabolic disarray – yet hold the frequency and duration of such occasions to a level consistent to a predominance of metabolic order. And if you indulge like me when you vacation, you will most certainly feel the return of metabolic disarray.

Just be warned that during your vacation, many of the forgotten nightmares of obesity may return with a vengeance. The wonderful lethargy, drowsiness, headaches, churning stomach, persistent hunger, gas, and diarrhea (to name a few) may come back to haunt you. But boy, is that chocolate cream pie a real treat.

I view the return of these simple ailments and discomforts as a blessing in disguise. Because after 48 hours (and sometimes only after 24 hours) of experiencing such gifts of carbohydrates, I am most ready to end my vacation. It certainly reminds me of why I need to remain on a low-carb plan in the long haul.

I can almost promise you that you will gain weight over a vacation period. Initially, because the abrupt increase in insulin levels causes water retention, and secondly because you are again a fat-producing and fat-saving machine. But I can also assure you that it comes off quickly once you return to ketosis. And remember, ketosis will not return (and insulin-derived hunger will not subside) until about 48 hours have elapsed from the time you stopped vacationing and returned to your low-carb plan. Man, is that a long 48 hours.

Fundamentals for Lasting Success

A low-carb plan is yours for life. A low-carb plan should be your life. A low-carb plan may very well mean your life. I leave you with simple rules for a life of success on any low-carb plan. Abide by them, and health and vitality will be yours once again!

The *Golden Rule* of any low-carb plan:

Stay in ketosis more often than not.

The *Silver Rules* of any low-carb plan:

Use your ketostix.
Don't limit the amount you eat. That is, eat to satisfaction.
Never count calories or fat.
Never fast to lose weight.

The *Bronze Rules* of any low-carb plan:

Eat a variety of foods.
Do not lump your daily allowance of carbohydrates in one meal.
Take a vacation once in a while.

CHAPTER 8

What You Can and Can't Eat on a Low-Carb Plan

It should be all too obvious to you that a low-carb plan is one sinfully delectable way to lose weight and keep it off for good. You'll suddenly find others observing your eating habits, shaking their heads in amazement, and wondering out loud how you can possibly remain so trim on such feastly foods. With a smile and a shrug, you can now offer that calories and fat simply don't affect your weight in the slightest ... and mean every word of it.

Menu of the Gods

In this chapter, you will find four basic food lists categorized by relative factors of consumption ... factors vital to your success on any low-carb plan. These categories are (1) foods that can be consumed with virtually no restriction to quantity, (2) foods that should be approached with some level of carbohydrate awareness, (3) foods that must be strictly proportioned when consumed, and (4) foods permitted only during the pre-selected "vacation" periods of your personalized low-carb plan.

You will notice that these lists identify foods in the most general of terms. You will also notice that brand names, many prepared dishes, and most ethnic foods are not addressed. Both of these, I'm afraid, are by design. A food list of this sort would easily become a book by itself, and indeed, many such books are available on the market today. So use this chapter for general guidance, but refer to a comprehensive "counter" whenever a question of carbohydrate content arises.

Remember, the setpoint for your fat-producing insulin switch leaves little room for guessing. So please don't guess! I also caution you never to assume carbohydrate equivalency between brands of identical foods. Always read the nutritional information provided on the food packaging. The smallest addition of flour, starch, corn syrup, fructose, or sugar can make one brand taboo while a competitor's brand may be allowed. For simplicity of reference, I have repeated foods listed on the 2-4 week menu of Chapter 6.

Foods Of Unlimited Quantity

These are foods that are so low or essentially absent of carbohydrates[1] that you needn't concern yourself as to how much or how often you consume them. Enjoy!

- beef[2] (steaks, roast, ribs, hamburgers, etc.)

- pork[2] (chops, roast, ribs, sausage, ham, bacon, etc.)

- lamb[2] (chops, roast, etc.)

- seafood[3] (fish, lobster, crab, shrimp, caviar, etc.)

- poultry/fowl[4] (chicken, turkey, duck, etc.)

- pressed meats (bologna, salami, cold cuts, pepperoni, wieners, hot dogs, etc.)

- eggs[5]

- cheese[6]

- cream cheese[6]

- butter[7]

- cooking oil

- salad dressing[6]

- mayonnaise[6,8]

- sour cream[6]

- heavy or double cream[9]

- real whipped cream

- mustard

- herbs and seasoning

- hot sauce

- vinegar

- pork rinds

- artificial sweeteners

- sugar-free gelatin

- sugar-free chewing gum[10]

- tea

- coffee

- diet soda

- sugar-free drinks and punch

- water (of course, including flavored seltzers)

Numbered Notes

1. When you prepare a food dish in which one or more ingredient isn't found on this list, do it with obsessive carbohydrate restriction in mind. For example, if you prepare taco meat, leave out the maize. If you prepare chili, leave out both the thickener and the beans.

2. There are of course many other types of meats that aren't shown, like venison, frogs legs, and escargot (to name a few). The rule of thumb is, if it used to fly, walk, hop, crawl, slither, or swim ... go for it.

3. Clams, oysters, scallops, and the like contain more than just a little carbohydrates, so they are not to be considered part of this list.

4. Leave the skin on if you wish!

5. Drop any remnants of concern you may have about consuming cholesterol-laden foods. On a low-carb plan, it is simply not an issue.

6. Avoid "diet", "low-calorie", and "low-fat" labels like the plague. They always contain more carbohydrates than the real thing.

7. Stay away from diet spreads. Why use margarine when butter is yours for the taking?

8. Beware of certain brands. Some actually add sugar!

9. No non-dairy creamers in your coffee or tea. What a shame.

10. I have found that some sugar-free things (like certain chewing gums and breath mints) play

havoc on my stomach. I don't know what the offending ingredient is, but I'm thinking that this is a good example of a food intolerance (as discussed in Chapter 4).

Foods Of Moderation

These are foods that have varying but relatively small amounts of carbohydrates per typical serving. Ration these on a daily basis. Some have so few carbohydrates that they almost belong on the previous list. They're not, so treat them accordingly.

- lettuce

- cabbage

- carrots

- radishes

- tomatoes

- mushrooms

- string beans

- celery

- watercress

- cucumbers

- olives

- dill pickles

- onions

- garlic

- green peppers

- thin, oily gravy

- bouillon or broth soup (no thick soups or noodles)

- cocktail sauce

- soy sauce

- tartar sauce

- cottage cheese

- cheese spreads

Foods Of Caution

I use the word "caution" because one standard portion of some of these foods would alone be enough to flip that fat-producing insulin switch back on. And where one serving may not do it, the carbohydrate content of most of these foods is deceptively low enough to prompt consumption without taking into consideration the daily accumulation of carbohydrates from the "moderation" menu.

Because these foods must be watched with the utmost of care, I have offered approximate carbohydrate values for the lot. And I emphasize the word approximate. These values are for general reference only. Always, always read the nutritional labels!

- light bread[1]
    - 6-11 gr/slice

- small dinner rolls
    - 6-10 gr/each

- croutons[2]
    - 7-9 gr/handful

- meat spreads
    - 3-5 gr/tbsp

- peanut butter
    - 2-5 gr/tbsp

- thick gravy
  2-5 gr/4 tbsps

- ketchup
  2-5 gr/tbsp

- horseradish
  2-5 gr/tbsp

- steak sauce
  3-5 gr/tbsp

- taco sauce
  3-5 gr/tbsp

- worcestershire sauce
  1-4 gr/tbsp

- barbecue sauce
  4-10 gr/tbsp

- pizza sauce
  6-12 gr/4 tbsps

- spaghetti sauce
  9-20 gr/8 tbsps

- salsa
  4-6 gr/4 tbsps

- asparagus
    2 gr/spear

- beets
    4 gr each

- broccoli
    7 gr/cup

- brussel sprouts
    5 gr/half-cup

- cauliflower
    6 gr/cup

- eggplant
    9 gr/cup

- mustard greens
    6 gr/cup

- okra
    9 gr/cup

- green peppers
    4 gr/cup

- avocado
    7 gr/half

- grapefruit
    10 gr/half

- strawberries
    6 gr/four

- grapes
    5 gr/ten

- lemon
    2 gr/wedge

- peach
    5 gr/half

- apples
    10 gr/half

- oranges
    10 gr/half

- almonds
    6 gr/small handful

- macadamia nuts
    4 gr/small handful

- pistachio nuts (unshelled)
    6 gr/small handful

- brazil nuts
    4 gr/small handful

- cashews
    5 gr/small handful

- popcorn (popped)
    6 gr/cup

- cooking wine
    1-5 gr/4 tbsps

- wine and champagne[3]
    2-4 gr/half cup

- light beer
    2-12 gr/12 oz

- vegetable juice
    6-8 gr/cup

- soy flour
    10 gr/half cup

Numbered Notes

1.   Bakeries aren't the least bit interested in making a low-carbohydrate bread. They do, however, specifically cater to the ill-advised public who demand a low-fat, low-calorie bread. So it is strictly coincidence that "diet" breads are also

lower in carbohydrates per slice than their non-diet counterparts. The primary reason is because they are cut thinner and are much less dense.

2.   Why not make your own croutons with light bread bits and lots of seasoned cooking oil?

3.   Beware sweet wines and champagnes. Some pack carbohydrate punches ten times that of the above-listed value.

Vacation Foods

These are the foods that you must absolutely and positively avoid in order to keep the fat-producing insulin switch in the "off" position. They should only be considered when you vacation periodically from your low-carb plan (as discussed in Chapter 7). Again, limit your vacations to less than 15 per year, and never for more than 48 hours per vacation.

- rice

- pasta

- spaghetti

- macaroni

- beans (pinto, navy, brown, lima, etc.)

- thick soups

- soups with noodles

- potatoes

- corn

- peas

- flour/meal (wheat, rye, corn, white, almond, matzo, etc.)

- cornstarch

- potato starch

- pancakes

- waffles

- cakes

- pies

- pastries

- muffins

- croissants

- doughnuts

- cookies

- sweet rolls

- pretzels

- bagels

- sugar[1]

- candy

- chocolate

- chewing gum

- mints

- breakfast cereals

- breakfast bars

- grain bars

- yogurt

- ice cream

- sherbet

- pudding

- jam

- jelly

- preserves

- honey

- syrup

- chips

- snack crackers

- relish

- sweet pickles

- bananas

- pears

- milk

- milk flavorings

- cocoa mix

- sport drinks

- fruit drinks

- regular soda

- regular beer

- fruit juice, fresh or concentrated

- spirits and liquors

Numbered Notes

1.   Watch out for cold medications and lozenges. Many use sugar to make them palatable to children, and tempting for adults.